Table of Contents

Introduction

Fatty liver disease means you have extra fat in your liver. You might hear your doctor call it hepatic steatosis.

Heavy drinking makes you more likely to get it. Over time, too much alcohol leads to a buildup of fat inside your liver cells. This makes it harder for your liver to work.

But you can get fatty liver disease even if you don't drink a lot of alcohol.

Fatty liver is the accumulation of triglycerides and other fats in the liver cells. The amount of fatty acid in the liver depends on the balance between the processes of delivery and removal. In some patients, fatty liver may be accompanied by hepatic inflammation and liver cell death (steatohepatitis).

Fat in the liver typically develops when a person consumes more fat and sugars than his or her body can handle. This is more common in people who are overweight or obese but can also occur in adults with healthy body weights. If fat builds up to more than 5% of the liver, then the liver is considered to be a fatty liver. Although having this condition may not cause any immediate harm, there is a concern that extra fat in the liver might make the liver vulnerable to further injury such as inflammation and scarring.

Non-alcoholic fatty liver disease (NAFLD) is a liver disease affecting people who drink little to no alcohol. As the name implies, the main characteristics of NAFLD is too much fat stored in liver cells. NAFLD is the most common liver disease in Canada affecting about 20% of Canadians.

It tends to develop in people who are overweight or obese, particularly if they have lot of fat around the middle of their body (waist). It can also develop in a person whose body weight is in the healthy weight range, but who typically eats a lot of sugary and fatty foods and who has extra fat around the waist.

NAFLD has shown to be strongly associated with metabolic syndrome—a health disorder characterized by a group of risk factors (large waist circumference, high blood pressure, high blood sugar levels, high cholesterol, and abnormal amounts of lipids in the blood) that greatly increase the risk of many chronic illnesses.

Fatty liver occurs when too much fat builds up in liver cells. Although it is normal to have a tiny amount of fat in these cells, the liver is considered fatty if more than 5% of it is fat.

While drinking too much alcohol can lead to fatty liver, in many cases it does not play a role.

A number of fatty liver conditions fall under the broad category of non-alcoholic liver disease (NAFLD), which is the most common liver disease in adults and children in Western countries..

Non-alcoholic fatty liver (NAFL) is the initial, reversible stage of liver disease. Unfortunately, it often goes undiagnosed. Over time, NAFL may lead to a more serious liver condition known as non-alcoholic steatohepatitis, or NASH.

Fatty liver is also known as hepatic steatosis. It happens when fat builds up in the liver. Having small amounts of fat in your liver is normal, but too much can become a health problem.

NASH involves greater fat accumulation and inflammation that damages the liver cells.This can lead to fibrosis, or scar tissue, as liver cells are repeatedly injured and die off.

Unfortunately, it is difficult to predict whether fatty liver will progress to NASH, which greatly increases the risk of cirrhosis (severe scarring that impairs liver function) and liver cancer.

NAFLD is also linked to an increased risk of other diseases, including heart disease, diabetes and kidney disease.

Your liver is the second largest organ in your body. It helps process nutrients from food and drinks and filters harmful substances from your blood.

Too much fat in your liver can cause liver inflammation, which can damage your liver and create scarring. In severe cases, this scarring can lead to liver failure.

When fatty liver develops in someone who drinks a lot of alcohol, it's known as alcoholic fatty liver disease (AFLD).

In someone who doesn't drink a lot of alcohol, it's known as non-alcoholic fatty liver disease (NAFLD). According to researchers in the World Journal of Gastroenterology, NAFLD affects up to 25 to 30 percent of people in the United States and Europe.

Symptoms of fatty liver
In many cases, fatty liver causes no noticeable symptoms. But you may feel tired or experience discomfort or pain in the upper right side of your abdomen.

Some people with fatty liver disease develop complications, including liver scarring. Liver scarring is known as liver fibrosis. If you develop severe liver fibrosis, it's known as cirrhosis.

Cirrhosis may cause symptoms such as:

- loss of appetite

- weight loss

- weakness

- fatigue

- nosebleeds

- itchy skin

- yellow skin and eyes

- web-like clusters of blood vessels under your skin

- abdominal pain

- abdominal swelling

- swelling of your legs

- breast enlargement in men

- confusion

Cirrhosis is a potentially life-threatening condition. Get the information you need to recognize and manage it.

Causes of fatty liver

Fatty liver develops when your body produces too much fat or doesn't metabolize fat efficiently enough. The excess fat is stored in liver cells, where it accumulates and causes fatty liver disease.

This build-up of fat can be caused by a variety of things.

For example, drinking too much alcohol can cause alcoholic fatty liver disease. This is the first stage of alcohol-related liver disease.

In people who don't drink a lot of alcohol, the cause

of fatty liver disease is less clear.

One or more of the following factors may play a role:

- obesity

- high blood sugar

- insulin resistance

- high levels of fat, especially triglycerides, in your blood

- Less common causes include:

- pregnancy

- rapid weight loss

- some types of infections, such as hepatitis C

- side effects from some types of medications, such as methotrexate (Trexall), tamoxifen (Nolvadex), amiodorone (Pacerone), and valproic acid (Depakote)

- exposure to certain toxins

Certain genes may also raise your risk of developing fatty liver.

Obesity: Obesity involves low-grade inflammation that may promote liver fat storage. It's estimated that 30–90% of obese adults have NAFLD, and it's increasing in children due to the childhood obesity epidemic.

Excess belly fat: Normal-weight people may develop fatty liver if they are "viscerally obese," meaning they carry too much fat around the waist.

Insulin resistance: Insulin resistance and high insulin levels have been shown to increase liver fat storage in people with type 2 diabetes and metabolic syndrome.

High intake of refined carbs: Frequent intake of refined carbs promotes liver fat storage, especially when high amounts are consumed by overweight or insulin-resistant individuals.

Sugary beverage consumption: Sugar-sweetened

beverages like soda and energy drinks are high in fructose, which has been shown to drive liver fat accumulation in children and adults.

Impaired gut health: Recent research suggests that having an imbalance in gut bacteria, problems with gut barrier function ("leaky gut") or other gut health issues may contribute to NAFLD development

Diagnosing of fatty liver
To diagnose fatty liver, your doctor will take your medical history, conduct a physical exam, and order one or more tests.

Medical history
If your doctor suspects that you might have fatty liver, they will likely ask you questions about:

- your family medical history, including any history of liver disease

- your alcohol consumption and other lifestyle habits

- any medical conditions that you might have

- any medications that you might take

- recent changes in your health

If you've been experiencing fatigue, loss of appetite, or other unexplained symptoms, let your doctor know.

Physical exam

To check for liver inflammation, your doctor may palpate or press on your abdomen.If your liver is enlarged, they might be able to feel it.

However, it's possible for your liver to be inflamed without being enlarged. Your doctor might not be able to tell if your liver is inflamed by touch.

Blood tests

In many cases, fatty liver disease is diagnosed after blood tests show elevated liver enzymes. For example, your doctor may order the alanine aminotransferase test (ALT) and aspartate aminotransferase test (AST) to check your liver enzymes.

These tests might be recommended if you've developed signs or symptoms of liver disease, or they might be ordered as part of routine blood work.

Elevated liver enzymes are a sign of liver inflammation. Fatty liver disease is one potential cause of liver inflammation, but it's not the only one.

If you test positive for elevated liver enzymes, your doctor will likely order additional tests to identify the cause of the inflammation.

Imaging studies

Your doctor may use one or more of the following

imaging tests to check for excess fat or other problems with your liver:

- ultrasound exam

- CT scan

- MRI scan

They might also order a test known as vibration-controlled transient elastography (VCTE, FibroScan). This test uses low-frequency sound waves to measure liver stiffness. It can help check for scarring.

Liver biopsy

A liver biopsy is considered the best way to determine the severity of liver disease.

During a liver biopsy, a doctor will insert a needle into your liver and remove a piece of tissue for examination. They will give you a local anesthetic to lessen the pain.

This test can help determine if you have fatty liver disease, as well as liver scarring.

Treatment for fatty liver

Currently, no medications have been approved to treat fatty liver disease. More research is needed to develop and test medications to treat this condition.

In many cases, lifestyle changes can help reverse fatty liver disease. For example, your doctor might advise you to:

- limit or avoid alcohol

- take steps to lose weight

- make changes to your diet

If you've developed complications, your doctor might recommend additional treatments. To treat cirrhosis, for example, they might prescribe:

- lifestyle changes

- medications

- surgery

- Cirrhosis can lead to liver failure. If you develop liver failure, you might need a liver transplant.

- Home remedies

- Lifestyle changes are the first-line treatment for fatty liver disease. Depending on your current condition and lifestyle habits, it might help to:

- lose weight

- reduce your alcohol intake

- eat a nutrient-rich diet that's low in excess calories, saturated fat, and trans fats

- get at least 30 minutes of exercise most days of the week

According to the Mayo Clinic, some evidence suggests that vitamin E supplements might help prevent or treat liver damage caused by fatty liver disease. However, more research is needed. There are some health risks associated with consuming too much vitamin E.

Always talk to your doctor before you try a new supplement or natural remedy. Some supplements or natural remedies might put stress on your liver or interact with medications you're taking.

Diet for fatty liver disease

If you have fatty liver disease, your doctor might encourage you to adjust your diet to help treat the condition and lower your risk of complications. For example, they might advise you to do the following:

- Eat a diet that's rich in plant-based foods, including fruits, vegetables, legumes, and whole grains.

- Limit your consumption of refined carbohydrates, such as sweets, white rice, white bread, other refined grain products.

- Limit your consumption of saturated fats, which are found in red meat and many other animal products.

- Avoid trans fats, which are present in many processed snack foods.

- Avoid alcohol.

Your doctor may encourage you to cut calories from your diet to lose weight. Learn more about some of the other dietary changes that might help you manage fatty liver disease.

Dietary Strategies for Getting Rid of Fatty Liver

There are several things you can do to get rid of fatty liver, including losing weight and cutting back on carbs. What's more, certain foods can help you lose liver fat.

Lose Weight and Avoid Overeating If Overweight or Obese

Weight loss is one of the best ways to reverse fatty liver if you are overweight or obese.

In fact, weight loss has been shown to promote loss of liver fat in adults with NAFLD, regardless of whether the weight loss was achieved by making dietary changes alone or in combination with weight loss surgery or exercise.

In a three-month study of overweight adults, reducing calorie intake by 500 calories per day led to an 8% loss of body weight, on average, and a significant decrease in fatty liver score.

What's more, it appears that the improvements in liver fat and insulin sensitivity may persist even if some of the weight is regained.

Cut Back on Carbs, Especially Refined Carbs

It may seem as though the most logical way to address fatty liver would be to cut back on dietary fat.

However, researchers report only about 16% of liver fat in people with NAFLD comes from dietary fat. Rather, most liver fat comes from fatty acids in their blood, and about 26% of liver fat is formed in a process called de novo lipogenesis (DNL).

During DNL, excess carbs are converted into fat. The rate at which DNL occurs increases with high intakes of fructose-rich foods and beverages.

In one study, obese adults who consumed a diet high in calories and refined carbs for three weeks experienced a 27% increase in liver fat, on average, even though their weight only increased by 2%.

Studies have shown that consuming diets low in refined carbs may help reverse NAFLD. These include low-carb, Mediterranean and low-glycemic index diets.

In one study, liver fat and insulin resistance decreased significantly more when people consumed a Mediterranean diet than when they consumed a low-fat, high-carb diet, even though weight loss was similar on both diets.

Although both Mediterranean and very low-carb diets have been shown to reduce liver fat on their own, one study that combined them showed very impressive results.

In this study, 14 obese men with NAFLD followed a Mediterranean ketogenic diet. After 12 weeks, 13 of the men experienced reductions in liver fat, including three who achieved complete resolution of fatty liver.

Include Foods That Promote Loss of Liver Fat
In addition to cutting back on carbs and avoiding excess calorie intake, there are certain foods and beverages that may be beneficial for fatty liver:

Monounsaturated fats: Research suggests that eating foods high in monounsaturated fatty acids like olive oil, avocados and nuts may promote liver fat loss.

Whey protein: Whey protein has been shown to reduce liver fat by up to 20% in obese women. In addition, it may help lower liver enzyme levels and provide other benefits in people with more advanced liver disease.

Green tea: One study found that antioxidants in green tea called catechins helped decrease liver fat and inflammation in people with NAFLD.

Soluble fiber: Some research suggests that consuming 10–14 grams of soluble fiber daily may help reduce liver fat, decrease liver enzyme levels and increase insulin sensitivity.

Types of fatty liver disease
There are two main types of fatty liver disease:

nonalcoholic and alcoholic.

Nonalcoholic fatty liver disease (NAFLD) includes simple nonalcoholic fatty liver, nonalcoholic steatohepatitis (NASH), and acute fatty liver of pregnancy (AFLP).

Alcoholic fatty liver disease (AFLD) includes simple AFLD and alcoholic steatohepatitis (ASH).

Nonalcoholic fatty liver disease (NAFLD)
Nonalcoholic fatty liver disease (NAFLD) occurs when fat builds up in the liver of people who don't drink a lot of alcohol.

If you have excess fat in your liver and no history of heavy alcohol use, your doctor may diagnose you with NAFLD.

If there's no inflammation or other complications along with the build-up of fat, the condition is known as simple nonalcoholic fatty liver.

Nonalcoholic steatohepatitis (NASH)

Nonalcoholic steatohepatitis (NASH) is a type of NAFLD. It occurs when a build-up of excess fat in the liver is accompanied by liver inflammation.

If you have excess fat in your liver, your liver is inflamed, and you have no history of heavy alcohol use, your doctor may diagnose you with NASH.

When left untreated, NASH can cause scarring of your liver. In severe cases, this can lead to cirrhosis and liver failure.

Acute fatty liver of pregnancy (AFLP)

Acute fatty liver of pregnancy (AFLP) is a rare but serious complication of pregnancy. The exact cause is unknown.

When AFLP develops, it usually appears in the third trimester of pregnancy. If left untreated, it poses serious health risks to the mother and growing baby.

If you're diagnosed with AFLP, your doctor will want to deliver your baby as soon as possible. You might need to receive follow-up care for several days after you give birth.

Your liver health will likely return to normal within a few weeks of giving birth.

Alcoholic fatty liver disease (ALFD)
Drinking a lot of alcohol damages the liver. When it's damaged, the liver can't break down fat properly. This can cause fat to build up, which is known as alcoholic fatty liver.

Alcoholic fatty liver disease (ALFD) is the earliest stage of alcohol-related liver disease.

If there's no inflammation or other complications along with the build-up of fat, the condition is known as simple alcoholic fatty liver.

Alcoholic steatohepatitis (ASH)

Alcoholic steatohepatitis (ASH) is a type of AFLD. It happens when a build-up of excess fat in the liver is accompanied by liver inflammation. This is also known as alcoholic hepatitis.

If you have excess fat in your liver, your liver is inflamed, and you drink a lot of alcohol, your doctor may diagnose you with ASH.

If it's not treated properly, ASH can cause scarring of your liver. Severe liver scarring is known as cirrhosis. It can lead to liver failure.

To treat alcoholic fatty liver, it's important to avoid alcohol. If you have alcoholism, or alcohol use disorder, your doctor may recommend counseling or other treatments. Read more about the effects that alcohol can have on your body.

Exercise That Can Help Reduce Liver Fat

Physical activity can be an effective way to

decrease liver fat.

Studies have shown that engaging in endurance exercise or resistance training several times a week can significantly reduce the amount of fat stored in liver cells, regardless of whether weight loss occurs.

In a four-week study, 18 obese adults with NAFLD who exercised for 30–60 minutes five days per week experienced a 10% decrease in liver fat, even though their body weight remained stable.

High-intensity interval training (HIIT) has also been shown to be beneficial for decreasing liver fat.

In a study of 28 people with type 2 diabetes, performing HIIT for 12 weeks led to an impressive 39% reduction in liver fat.

However, even lower-intensity exercise can be effective at targeting liver fat. According to a large Italian study, it appears that how much you exercise is most important.

In that study, 22 diabetics who worked out twice per

week for 12 months had similar reductions in liver fat and abdominal fat, regardless of whether their exercise intensity was considered low-to-moderate or moderate-to-high.

Since working out regularly is important for reducing liver fat, choosing something you like doing and can stick with is your best strategy.

Supplements That May Improve Fatty Liver
Results from several studies suggest that certain vitamins, herbs and other supplements may help reduce liver fat and decrease the risk of liver disease progression.

However, in most cases, experts say that further research is required to confirm this.

In addition, it's important to speak with your doctor before taking any supplements, especially if you are taking medication.

Milk Thistle

Milk thistle, or silymarin, is an herb known for its liver-protecting effects..

Some studies have found that milk thistle, alone or in combination with vitamin E, may help reduce insulin resistance, inflammation and liver damage in people with NAFLD.

In a 90-day study of people with fatty liver, the group who took a silymarin-vitamin E supplement and followed a low-calorie diet experienced twice the reduction in liver size as the group who followed the diet without taking the supplement.

The dosages of milk thistle extract used in these studies were 250–376 mg per day.

However, although experts believe that milk thistle shows promise for use in NAFLD, they feel that more studies are needed to confirm its effectiveness for both short- and long-term use.

Berberine

Berberine is a plant compound that has been shown to significantly reduce blood sugar, insulin and cholesterol levels, along with other health markers.

Several studies also suggest that it may benefit people with fatty liver.

In a 16-week study, 184 people with NAFLD reduced their calorie intake and exercised for at least 150 minutes per week. One group took berberine, one took an insulin-sensitizing drug and the other group took no supplement or medication.

Those taking 500 mg of berberine, three times per day at meals, experienced a 52% reduction in liver fat and greater improvements in insulin sensitivity and other health markers than the other groups.

Researchers say that despite these encouraging results, further studies are needed to confirm berberine's effectiveness for NAFLD.

Omega-3 Fatty Acids

Omega-3 fatty acids have been credited with many health benefits. The long-chain omega-3s EPA and DHA are found in fatty fish, such as salmon, sardines, herring and mackerel.

Several studies have shown that taking omega-3s may improve liver health in adults and children with fatty liver.

In a controlled study of 51 overweight children with NAFLD, the group who took DHA had a 53% reduction in liver fat, compared to 22% in the placebo group. The DHA group also lost more belly fat and fat around the heart.

Furthermore, in a study of 40 adults with fatty liver, 50% of those who took fish oil in addition to making dietary changes had reductions in liver fat, while 33% experienced a complete resolution of fatty liver.

The dosages of omega-3 fatty acids used in these studies were 500–1,000 mg per day in children and 2–4 grams per day in adults.

Although all the studies above used fish oil, you can get the same benefits by consuming fish high in omega-3 fats several times a week.

Importantly, these studies show that certain supplements appear to enhance the effects of lifestyle changes. Taking them without following a healthy diet and exercising regularly will likely have little effect on liver fat.

Risk factors

Drinking high amounts of alcohol puts you at increased risk of developing fatty liver.

You may also be at heightened risk if you:

- are obese

- have insulin resistance

- have type 2 diabetes

- have polycystic ovary syndrome

- are pregnant

- have a history of certain infections, such as hepatitis C

- take certain medications, such as methotrexate (Trexall), tamoxifen (Nolvadex), amiodorone (Pacerone), and valproic acid (Depakote)

- have high cholesterol levels

- have high triglyceride levels

- have high blood sugar levels

- have metabolic syndrome

If you have a family history of fatty liver disease, you're more likely to develop it yourself.

Stages of fatty liver

Fatty liver can progress through four stages:

Simple fatty liver. There is a build-up of excess fat in the liver.

Steatohepatitis. In addition to excess fat, there is inflammation in the liver.

Fibrosis. Inflammation in the liver has caused scarring.

Cirrhosis. Scarring of the liver has become widespread.

Cirrhosis is a potentially life-threatening condition that can cause liver failure. It may be irreversible. That's why it's so important to prevent it from developing in the first place.

To help stop fatty liver from progressing and causing complications, follow your doctor's recommended treatment plan.

Prevention

To prevent fatty liver and its potential complications,

it's important to follow a healthy lifestyle.

- Limit or avoid alcohol.

- Maintain a healthy weight.

- Eat a nutrient-rich diet that's low in saturated fats, trans fats, and refined carbohydrates.

- Take steps to control your blood sugar, triglyceride levels, and cholesterol levels.

- Follow your doctor's recommended treatment plan for diabetes, if you have it.

- Aim for at least 30 minutes of exercise most days of the week.

- Taking these steps can also help improve your overall health.

Outlook

In many cases, it's possible to reverse fatty liver through lifestyle changes. These changes may help prevent liver damage and scarring.

The condition can cause inflammation, damage to your liver, and potentially irreversible scarring if it's not treated. Severe liver scarring is known as cirrhosis.

If you develop cirrhosis, it increases your risk of liver cancer and liver failure. These complications can be fatal.

For the best outcome, it's important to follow your doctor's recommended treatment plan and practice an overall healthy lifestyle.

Fatty Liver Diet: Menu, Plan, Recipes

Table covered in healthy food, including salmon, broccoli, pecans, and spinach

Eating the wrong foods can damage your liver as much as alcohol. When your body stores too much liver fat, the result is inflammation, scarring, and permanent damage. Even if things don't go as far as liver failure, nonalcoholic fatty liver disease (NAFLD) places you at much higher risk for several serious chronic conditions. And it affects as many as 100 million Americans, making it the most common chronic liver disease.

NAFLD isn't well understood, but there are some things we do know. We know its risk factors include metabolic syndrome, sleep apnea, type 2 diabetes, heart disease, high triglyceride levels, and obesity. While you can't do anything about many of those risk factors, those you can influence are almost entirely linked to a healthy diet. That's why the most effective therapeutic method of battling NAFLD is no more complicated than having a fatty liver diet plan.

Fatty Liver Foods to Avoid
Added sugars contribute to hypertension and excess fat in the liver. Sugar can be found in

obvious places like sweetened beverages, but it's also lurking in most processed foods. It almost goes without saying, but this includes alcoholic beverages, which are known to contribute to the development of fatty liver disease and cirrhosis.

Furthermore, a fatty liver diet menu will heavily restrict the consumption of refined grains. Having been stripped of their fibrous content, refined grains are rapidly digested by the body. The result is a change in insulin resistance that's almost on par with eating raw sugar. Do your best to avoid simple carbohydrates like white bread, white rice, potatoes, rice milk, rice crackers, and cornflakes.

Foods to Seek Out

Broccoli may help prevent buildup of fat in the liver, and clinical studies have found garlic powder can help reduce body weight for people with fatty liver disease. Additionally, research suggests omega-3 fatty acids are good for improving cholesterol problems. Omega 3 is found in sardines, walnuts, salmon, and similar fresh fish.

If you're trying to lose weight, then stick to foods that are lower on the glycemic index, like vegetables. In place of simple carbs, switch to complex carbs. Whole grain bread, oatmeal, and wheat bran cereal are good choices.

Foods to Eat in Moderation

No human studies have connected NAFLD and the consumption of saturated fat. Because triglyceride levels can actually increase with reduced-fat diets and high levels of carbohydrate consumption are associated with liver inflammation, you'll want to eat saturated fat in moderation rather than eliminating it entirely.

But don't get your saturated fats from low-quality sources, like processed foods. Good sources of saturated fats include things like fatty meats, dairy, avocado, and most types of nut.

Planning For Fatty Liver Disease

You may have noticed that the fatty liver diet menu is composed of classic diet foods. That's because for most people the best way to take on NAFLD is losing weight.But regular exercise can make dietary changes far more effective than dietary changes alone. If you or a loved one are making dietary changes in the interests of health, don't forget to put some regular activity on the menu as well.

Non-alcoholic fatty liver disease (NAFLD) is now the most common cause of chronic liver disease worldwide and will have a major impact on the health care requirements of many countries in the future. NAFLD can progress to cirrhosis, liver cancer and liver failure. These are the reasons I have done a lot of research into the diet and nutritional therapies that can reverse the pathology of NAFLD.

The liver possesses remarkable properties of repair

and renewal and it is possible to completely reverse NAFLD if it is detected early enough. We are seeing NAFLD in a much younger population and it is not uncommon in overweight children. This is worrying because the earlier in life you develop a fatty liver, the more likely you are to develop complications.

I have developed a very specific way of eating, which is designed to:

- Reduce the fat in the liver

- Minimize liver damage

- Improve the function of insulin

- Make weight loss easier

This is not a low-fat low-calorie diet, and unlike those old fashioned diets, will not leave you hungry and tired. It is not a high protein diet either but rather provides you with first class protein regularly throughout the day, along with plenty of vegetables and some good fats.

Enjoy this way of eating, as your liver will definitely thank you for it!

With your meals it is ideal to include:

Raw plant food, especially raw vegetables.A maximum of 2 pieces of fruit daily are allowed while you are trying to lose weight. Most fruits are fairly high in sugar.Vegetables contain very little sugar, therefore you can eat unlimited quantities.

Cooked vegetables of different varieties including some starchy vegetables (except potatoes); this will compensate for the fact that you will not be eating bread, biscuits and sugary desserts.

First class protein from one or more of the following choices –

- Any seafood, canned or fresh (not smoked or deep -fried)

- Poultry

- Lean fresh red meats

- Eggs – organic or free range

- Legumes (beans, chickpeas or lentils) & raw nuts & seeds

- Protein powder – make sure it does not contain sugar; ideally use Synd-X Slimming Protein powder which is sweetened with the herb stevia. You can use this powder to make delicious smoothies.

Take a good liver tonic to support your liver function

Livatone Plus contains all the nutrients your liver requires for efficient phase 1 and 2 detoxification. It also contains the herb St Mary's Thistle, which helps to repair damaged liver cells.

Increase glutathione production

Glutathione is your liver's most powerful detoxifier and it is strongly anti-inflammatory. If you have a fatty liver you need more of it. N-acetyl cysteine is a precursor of glutathione and is known to raise blood levels powerfully.Eating sulfur rich foods also helps with glutathione; examples include eggs, cabbage, broccoli and garlic.

Extra Tip: Satisfy your hunger

You may eat enough to satisfy your natural hunger at every meal and snack. Those who work in occupations requiring high physical exertion or those who do a lot of sport will need to eat larger amounts. Listen to your body and follow your natural instincts when it comes to the amount of food you need to eat to feel satisfied and happy. It is not how much you eat that counts, it is what you are eating that is so important for your liver and insulin levels.

Quick easy healthy snacks

Healthy in between meal snacks may include –

Canned seafood (sardines, salmon, mackerel, crab meat or tuna) – one small can mixed with the juice of ½ a fresh lemon or 1 Tbsp of natural yoghurt and fresh chopped herbs.

A protein smoothie made with coconut milk or almond milk and 3 tablespoons fresh or frozen berries.

Raw nuts and seeds of any variety by themselves, or with 1 piece of fresh fruit. Fresh nuts are best and you can add salt to them if desired. Use one handful of nuts maximum.

Raw vegetables - good examples are carrot, cucumber, zucchini, or celery sticks, or broccoli florets dipped into tahini, hummus or freshly mashed avocado.

Raw fruit – one to two pieces of fruit by itself - or with 10 raw nuts or plain yoghurt.

Avocado Dip or Bean Dip with sticks of raw vegetables or par-steamed vegetables such as broccoli, cauliflower.

A raw vegetable juice – one glass full. Raw juices are an excellent source of highly concentrated vitamins, minerals and antioxidants. My book Raw Juices can Save your Life contains numerous raw juice recipes.

Remember to stay away from or minimize the following danger foods–

Sugar and candy; some cheap chocolates contain hydrogenated vegetable oils which are most unhealthy. If you do indulge in a little chocolate the best types are dark chocolate with a minimum of 70 percent cocoa solids.

Foods containing flour.

"Diet foods" that claim to be slimming – they are usually low in fat and high in sugar or artificial sweeteners, eg. Diet yogurts, diet jams, diet ice-cream, diet sodas, etc; These diet foods are not slimming; they are very fattening.

Fried snacks – such as potato chips, tortilla chips, pretzels, crackers, etc.

Pizza

Fried take away foods.

Biscuits – both sweet and savoury varieties, as they contain flour, hydrogenated vegetable oils, and if sweet will be high in sugar.

Crumpets, muffins, bagels, white bread and donuts.

CRUSTLESS QUICHE CUPS

Eggs have gotten a bad rap in recent years, but they are full of protein and essential vitamins and minerals. Whip them up with some veggies for this traditional breakfast favorite.

Serves 6

Ingridients

- Nonstick cooking spray

- 1 (10-ounce) package frozen chopped kale, or 2 cups chopped fresh

- 2 large eggs, plus 3 large egg whites

- ¼ cup chopped leek

- ¼ cup chopped sun-dried tomato

- ¼ cup seeded and chopped yellow bell pepper

Steps

1. Preheat the oven to 350°F. Line a six-cup muffin pan with paper liners and spray with nonstick cooking spray.

2. If using frozen kale, microwave it for 2½ minutes on high, then drain away the excess liquid. Combine the eggs, egg whites, leek, sun-dried tomatoes, kale, and bell pepper in a

bowl and mix well. Divide the mixture equally among the prepared muffin cups.

Bake for 20 minutes, or until a knife comes out clean after being inserted in the center.

Note: These will stay fresh in the fridge for a few days, but they don't freeze well.

VEGETABLE FRITTATA

This Spanish-Italian dish is so versatile: it makes a great brunch; or you can cook it up for dinner and serve it with salad—and take leftovers for lunch the following day. No matter when you eat it, it's nutritious, filling, and flavorful.

Serves 4

Ingridients

- 2 large eggs, plus 4 large egg whites

- ¼ cup Parmesan cheese

- 1 teaspoon ground turmeric

- ½ cup seeded and chopped orange bell pepper

- ½ cup chopped red onion

- 1 teaspoon minced fresh garlic

- ½ teaspoon olive oil

- 2 cups washed and torn or chopped spinach

- Sea salt and freshly ground black pepper

Steps

Whisk the eggs and egg whites in a medium-size bowl. Add the Parmesan, turmeric, bell pepper, red onion, and garlic; mix lightly. Heat the olive oil in nonstick pan over medium heat and add the egg mixture. Then, add the spinach leaves on top of the egg mixture. When the frittata is partially cooked (the perimeter of the eggs can be easily lifted with a spatula), place a plate on top of the egg mixture and flip the pan. Then, slide the opposite side of the mixture back into the pan to cook further until the egg mixture has solidified. Season to taste with salt and pepper and cut into four equal wedges.

ZUCCHINI MUFFINS

Whip up a batch of these on the weekend and freeze half in individual bags for a healthy alternative to your morning pastry.

Makes 12 muffins

Ingridients

- Coconut oil cooking spray

- 1 cup walnuts or pecans

- 2 cups blanched almond flour

- 1 teaspoon ground allspice

- 1 teaspoon ground nutmeg

- 1 teaspoon ground cinnamon

- 1¼ teaspoons baking soda

- ½ teaspoon sea salt

- 1 teaspoon pure vanilla extract

- 2 large or 3 medium zucchini, grated

- 4 large eggs

- ⅓ cup applesauce

- ¼ cup extra-virgin coconut oil, melted

Steps

1. Preheat the oven to 350°F. Grease a twelve-cup muffin pan with coconut oil cooking spray.

2. Grind the walnuts or pecans in a food processor until coarse. Combine the ground nuts, almond flour, spices, baking soda, and salt in a small bowl.

3. Meanwhile, mix the vanilla, grated zucchini, eggs, applesauce, and coconut oil together in a large bowl. Add the dry ingredients to the wet ingredients and stir well to combine.

4. Divide the mixture equally among the prepared muffin cups and bake for 30 minutes. You'll know they're done when a knife or toothpick inserted into the center of a muffin comes out clean. They can be stored in the fridge for up to 5 days.

SHAVED BRUSSELS SPROUTS SALAD

This easy recipe shows off these little cruciferous veggies in their best light: dressed simply, the bright flavors really shine.

Serves 8

Ingridients

- 1¾ pounds Brussels sprouts, trimmed, outer leaves removed

- 5 tablespoons extra-virgin olive oil

- 12 medium-size shallots, thinly sliced (about 2 cups)

- 6 garlic cloves, thinly sliced

- 2 tablespoons freshly squeezed lemon juice

- Sea salt and freshly ground black pepper

Steps

1. Working in small batches, place the Brussels sprouts in the feeding tube of a food processor that has been fitted with a thin slicing disk and slice the sprouts. Alternatively, slice them by hand into thin slices.

2. Heat the olive oil in a large pot over medium heat and sauté the shallots until they're

almost translucent, about 3 minutes. Add the garlic and cook, stirring, for 1 minute, then add the Brussels sprouts. Increase the heat to medium-high and sauté the Brussels sprouts until tender, about 8 minutes. Stir in the lemon juice, then season to taste with salt and pepper. Transfer to a serving bowl.

MISO SOUP WITH SPINACH AND TOFU

Just like the soup at your favorite Japanese restaurant, this recipe is easy, light, and filled with the probiotic goodness of miso and all the health benefits of sea vegetables.

Serves 8

Ingridients

- 1 (12-ounce) block firm silken tofu

- 1 sheet nori (dried seaweed), cut into strips (about ¼ cup)

- 4 tablespoons white miso paste

- 4 green onions or scallions, thinly sliced

- 6 cups washed and torn or chopped spinach leaves

- 2 cups shredded carrot, for serving

- 2 cups shelled edamame, for serving

Steps

1. Wrap the block of tofu in two layers of paper towels and place it on a plate. Press down with your hands or a bowl to squeeze out any extra moisture, then cut the tofu into ¼- to ½-inch cubes.

2. Bring 4 cups of water to a simmer in a saucepan over medium heat, then add the nori and cook for 6 minutes.

3. In the meantime, whisk the miso paste in a bowl with some of the warm water from the

pot until it's smooth, then add it to the pot. Add the tofu cubes, green onions, and spinach, and cook for another minute, or until all the ingredients are heated through.

4. Remove the soup from the heat and ladle it into eight bowls. Top each portion with ¼ cup of shredded carrot and ¼ cup of edamame. Serve immediately.

SALMON CAKES

These simple cakes make a satisfying meal when paired with brown rice and roasted vegetables or your favorite salad.

Serves 4

Ingridients

- Nonstick cooking spray

- 1 tablespoon extra-virgin olive oil

- 1 small red onion, finely chopped

- 2 tablespoons dried parsley

- 15 ounces canned wild salmon, drained, or 1½ cups cooked wild-caught salmon

- 1 large egg, lightly beaten

- 1½ teaspoons Dijon mustard

- 1¾ cups rolled oats

- ½ teaspoon freshly ground black pepper

Steps

1. Preheat the oven to 450°F.Coat a baking sheet with nonstick cooking spray and set aside.

2. Heat 1 ½ teaspoons of the olive oil in a large, nonstick skillet over medium-high heat. Add the red onion and cook, stirring, until

softened, about 3 minutes. Stir in the parsley, then remove from the heat.

3. Place the salmon in a medium-size bowl and use a fork to flake it apart; remove any bones and skin. Add the egg and mustard and mix well, then add the onion mixture, oats, and pepper, mixing well. Shape the salmon mixture into eight patties, each about 2½ inches wide.

4. Heat the remaining 1½ teaspoons of olive oil in the pan over medium heat, add four salmon patties, and cook until their underside is golden, 2 to 3 minutes. Using a wide spatula, turn them over onto the prepared baking sheet. Repeat with the remaining patties.

5. Bake the salmon cakes until they're golden on top and heated through, 15 to 20 minutes. After cooking, pat off any excess oil with a paper towel.

GARLICKY TOFU

Tofu is a great source of plant-based protein, providing about 9 grams for every 3 ounces. Better yet, studies show that soy may help to alleviate symptoms of fatty liver. Pair that with inflammation -fighting garlic and you've got a meal your liver will cheer about!

Serves 4 to 6

Ingridients

- 1 (14-ounce) package extra-firm tofu

- 3 tablespoons olive oil

- 3 tablespoons crushed garlic

- Sea salt and freshly ground black pepper

Step

1. Remove the tofu from the package and drain the water. Pat dry with paper towel and cut into 1-inch cubes. Place the tofu in a large bowl with 2 tablespoons of the olive oil, the garlic, and salt and pepper to taste. Mix thoroughly. In a separate pan, heat the remaining tablespoon of olive oil for 1 to 2 minutes, then add the tofu mixture. Sauté until the tofu is browned on all sides, 5 to 6 minutes. Serve immediately.

SPINACH TURKEY MEATBALLS

Adding spinach to these meatballs increases both the nutrition and the flavor. These are great served over whole wheat or grain-free spaghetti or rice with a side of veggies.

Serves 4

Ingridients

- Olive oil cooking spray

- 2 cups washed baby spinach

- 1 pound lean ground turkey

- 2 garlic cloves, minced

- 1 small shallot, finely chopped

- 1 large egg, lightly beaten

- ¾ cup whole-grain bread crumbs

- ½ cup grated Parmesan cheese

- ½ teaspoon sea salt

- ¼ teaspoon freshly ground black pepper

Steps

2. Preheat the oven to 450°F. Lightly spray a large baking dish with olive oil cooking spray and set aside.

3. Place a steamer basket over simmering

water in a pot over medium heat and steam the baby spinach until it's wilted, 1 to 2 minutes. Let the spinach cool, squeeze out the water, and chop.

4. In a large bowl, combine the ground turkey, garlic, shallot, egg, bread crumbs, Parmesan, salt, pepper, and spinach; mix well. Use your hands to form the mixture into twelve equal-size meatballs.

5. Transfer the meatballs to the prepared baking dish and bake for 15 to 20 minutes, until the meatballs are golden brown and no longer pink inside.

CRISPY CHICKPEAS

These delicious bites are a great snack or topper for salads.

Serves 6 to 8

Ingridients

- 2 (15-ounce) cans chickpeas

- Olive oil

- Sea salt

- Paprika

- Ground cumin

Steps

1. Preheat the oven to 425°F.

2. Rinse and drain the chickpeas, then pat them dry. Place in a single layer on a rimmed baking sheet and lightly drizzle with olive oil. Roast until the chickpeas are dark and crunchy, 30 to 40 minutes.

3. Remove from the oven, sprinkle to taste with salt, paprika, and cumin, then roast for a few more minutes.

4. Remove from the oven and allow the chickpeas to cool before serving.They can be stored in an airtight container in the fridge for about 3 days.

CHICKEN SALAD

A healthier twist on this lunchtime favorite! Swap traditional mayo for Vegenaise, an egg-free spread that's high in omega-3s. With garlic, mustard, and celery, you won't notice any difference in the taste.

Serves 4

Ingridients

- 2 whole or 4 half chicken breasts, bone in, skin on

- Olive oil

- Kosher salt and freshly ground black pepper

- ½ cup Vegenaise

- ½ teaspoon Dijon mustard

- 1 teaspoon minced fresh garlic

- 1 cup diced celery (about 2 stalks)

- 1 cup green grapes, cut into quarters

Steps

1. Preheat the oven to 350°F.

2. Place the chicken breasts, skin side up, on a baking sheet, rub them with olive oil, and sprinkle generously with salt and pepper. Roast for 35 to 40 minutes, or until the chicken is cooked through.Set aside to cool.

3. When the chicken is cool, remove the meat from the bones and discard the skin and bones.

4. Dice the chicken into ¾-inch pieces and place in a bowl. Add the Vegenaise, mustard, garlic,

celery, and grapes, plus 1½ to 2 teaspoons of salt and 1 teaspoon of pepper or to taste. Toss well, then refrigerate until ready to serve.